Keto Recipes for Beginners

The Wholesome Yum Easy Keto Cookbook: 50 Simple Low Carb Recipes

by John Brady

Sommario

INTRODUCTION

Most people's expectations are to lose weight on this diet. However, the ketogenic diet focuses on whole health and supports all aspects, not just weight loss.

Ketogenic diets have significant benefits in various contexts. It has been shown to help control blood pressure and promote a healthy weight.

Originally designed to treat epilepsy, this diet takes advantage of ketosis, using ingredients to provide energy without using carbohydrates.

Great for keeping the body healthy, have immediate effects, keep insulin under control and thus prevent diabetes of different types.

This cookbook is designed for the less experienced, so I propose easy recipes, tasty and fast to start to dive into this wonderful world.

But I do not want to get lost in telling so many words, let's start cooking right away.

Are you ready?

Let's get started.

CHAPTER ONE

BREAKFAST

Keto Breakfast Burger

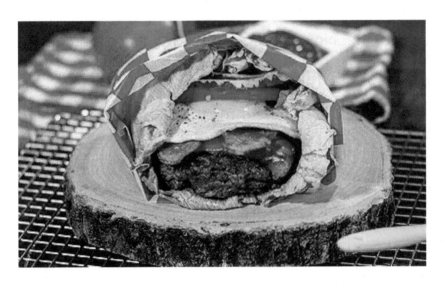

Prep Time: 13 Min | Cooking Time: 30 Min | Servings: 2

Ingredients

- 2 large Eggs
- 4 slices Bacon
- 4 oz. Sausage
- Salt and Pepper, to Taste

- 1 tbsp. Butter
- 2 oz. Pepper Jack Cheese

Directions

1. Preheat the oven to 400 F.
2. Spot bacon in the oven and bake for 20 to 25 minutes. Add the butter and set aside.
3. Cook the sausage balls on both sides. Add cheese and cover with a lid. Remove from the pan. Simmer the egg and place it on top.
4. Serve immediately and enjoy!

Nutritional Facts:

Calories: 654.5, Fat 55.9g, Carbohydrates 3g, Protein 31g

Keto Con Huevos

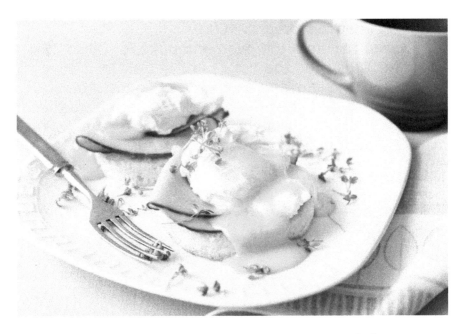

Prep Time: 11 Min | Cooking Time: 32 Min | Servings: 2

Ingredients

- 2 slices Bacon
- 3 Eggs
- 1 Jalapeno Pepper - de-seeded
- 1 Tomato
- 1 Avocado
- Salt and Pepper, to Taste
- 1/4 medium Onion
- 1/4 cup Cilantro, chopped
- 1 oz. Pork Rinds

Directions

1. Pour cold water over the bacon and let cook until done. Remove from heat and place on absorbent paper. Keep the fat in the pan.
2. Cook the pork rinds with the bacon fat and add the vegetables. When the onions are transparent, start mixing the cilantro. Add the scrambled eggs and cook, stirring once.
3. Trim the avocado into cubes and add it to the plate.
4. Serve immediately and enjoy!

Nutritional Facts:

Calories: 254, Fat 21.5g, Carbohydrates 2.5g, Protein 12.4g

Mini Baked Quiches

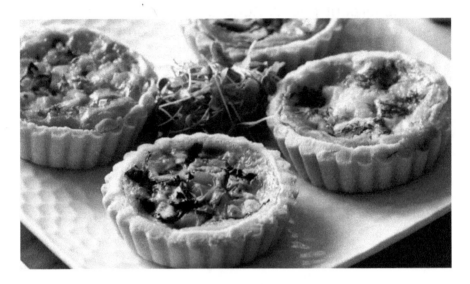

Prep Time: 13 Min | Cooking Time: 25 Min | Servings: 4

Ingredients

- 8 ounces white mushrooms, diced
- 1 teaspoon olive oil
- 4 ounces diced tomatoes
- 2 cloves minced garlic
- ¼ cup diced red onion
- 6 large eggs
- 1 tablespoon fresh chopped parsley
- ½ cup heavy cream
- Salt, to taste
- 1 cup shredded mozzarella cheese
- Pepper, to taste

Directions

1. Warm the oven to 350 degrees and grease a muffin pan with cooking spray.
2. In an enormous skillet, heat the oil over medium heat.
3. Add the mushrooms, tomatoes, red onion and garlic; then cook until tender, 6 to 8 minutes.
4. In a medium bowl, beat eggs, cream, parsley, salt and pepper until lightly combined.
5. Stir in the cooked vegetables and mozzarella.
6. Pour batter into prepared pan, filling cups evenly.
7. Bake for 22 to 25 minutes until the eggs are set and the top is lightly browned.
8. Let cool completely; then remove from the pot and refrigerate in an airtight container.

Nutritional Facts:

Calories: 329, Fat 26g, Cholesterol 342 mg, Carbohydrates 6g, Protein 18g

Pancakes with almonds and blueberries

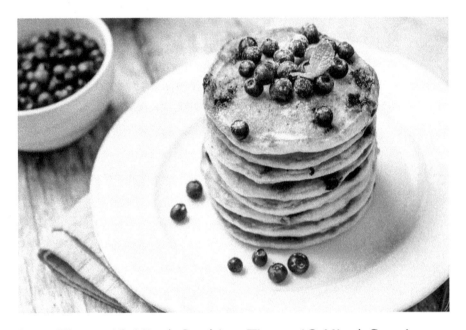

Prep Time: 12 Min | Cooking Time: 13 Min | Servings: 2

Ingredients

- 1 teaspoon baking powder
- 1 cup almond flour
- 3 large eggs
- Pinch salt

- 2 tablespoons unsweetened almond milk
- 2 tablespoons unsalted butter
- 1 tablespoon avocado oil
- ½ teaspoon vanilla extract
- ½ cup frozen blueberries

Directions

1. In a portable bowl, combine almond flour, baking powder and salt.
2. In a separate bowl, whisk together the eggs, vanilla extract and almond milk.
3. Spout the wet ingredients into the dry ingredients, beating and mix until smooth.
4. Heat and lightly grease a drip pan and pour batter onto the pan to make six 5-inch pancakes.
5. Sprinkle blueberries into the moist batter of each pancake, distributing them evenly over the pancakes.
6. Bake the pancakes until bubbles form on the surface of the dough.
7. Carefully flip the pancakes and cook until it turns golden brown on the bottom.
8. Slide the pancakes onto a plate and garnish them with butter to serve.

Nutritional Facts:

Calories: 614, Fat 54g, Cholesterol 310 mg, Carbohydrates 10g, Protein 22g

Poppy Seed Lemon Muffins

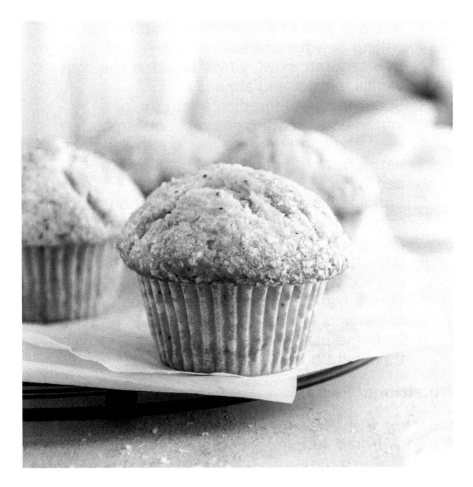

Prep Time: 11 Min | Cooking Time: 27 Min | Servings: 4

Ingredients

- 3/4 cup Almond Flour
- 2 large Eggs
- 1/3 cup Erythritol Powder
- 1/4 cup Heavy Cream
- 1/4 cup Flaxseed Meal
- 1/4 cup Salted Butter -melted
- 2 tbsp. Poppy Seeds
- 3 tbsp. Lemon Juice
- 1 tsp. Baking Powder
- Zest of 2 Lemons
- 1 tsp. Vanilla Extract

Directions

1. Preheat the oven to 350 F.
2. In a bowl, combine the erythritol, flax flour, almond flour and poppy seeds.
3. Add the eggs, melted butter and cream and mix until smooth. Then add the baking powder, vanilla, lemon juice and lemon zest. Mix until well blended.
4. Pour the batter evenly into 12 cupcake cups and bake for 18 to 20 minutes or until golden brown. Take it out from the heat and let it cool for about 10 minutes.
5. Cut and serve immediately.

Nutritional Facts:

Calories: 129, Fat 11.3g, Carbohydrates 1.5g, Protein 3.7g

Spiced Pumpkin French toast

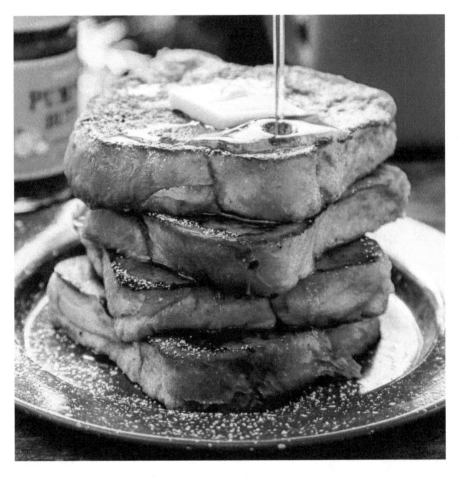

Prep Time: 13 Min | Cooking Time: 30 Min | Servings: 2

Ingredients

- 1 large Egg
- 4 slices Pumpkin Bread (refer to the recipe above)
- 2 tbsp. Cream
- 2 tbsp. Butter
- 1/2 tsp. Vanilla Extract
- 1/8 tsp. Orange Extract
- 1/4 tsp. Pumpkin Pie Spice

Directions

1. Let the bread dry overnight in an open-air. Stir in pumpkin pie spice, egg and orange extracts. Place the bread in the dough and let the pumpkin dough soak on both sides.
2. Warm the butter in a pan, and then add the marinated slices. Flip and cook until golden brown on each side.
3. Top with Keto Maple Syrup and enjoy!

Nutritional Facts:

Calories: 428, Fat 37.4g, Carbohydrates 6.8g, Protein 12g

Strawberries and Cream Shake

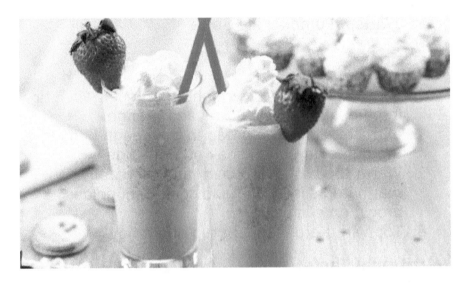

Prep Time: 5 Min | Cooking Time: 0 Min | Servings: 1

Ingredients

- ½ cup unsweetened almond milk
- ½ cup fresh strawberries
- ½ cup heavy cream
- 3 to 4 ice cubes
- 2 tablespoons sugar-free or unsweetened whipped cream, optional
- ½ teaspoon vanilla extract
- Liquid stevia extract, to taste

Directions

1. Wash the strawberries and cut the stems; then cut into large pieces.
2. In a blender combine the almond milk, cream and vanilla extract.
3. Add strawberries and ice cream, then mix until smooth.
4. Sweeten to taste with the liquid stevia, then mix until the mixture is smooth.
5. Pour into a glass and garnish with whipped cream to serve if desired.

Nutritional Facts:

Calories: 467, Fat 46g, Cholesterol 164 mg, Carbohydrates 8g, Protein 5g

Sweet Raspberry

Porridge

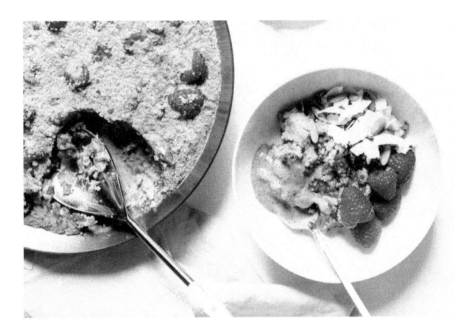

Prep Time: 5 Min | Cooking Time: 8 Min | Servings: 2

Ingredients

- ¼ cup ground flaxseed
- 2 cups unsweetened almond milk
- 8 to 10 drops liquid stevia extract, to taste
- ¼ cup coconut flour
- 1 teaspoon vanilla extract
- ⅔ cup fresh raspberries

Directions

1. In a portable saucepan, heat the almond milk over medium heat.
2. At the point that the almond milk comes to a boil, add the flax seeds and coconut flour until well combined.
3. Add the raspberries and cook until thickened, about 10 minutes.
4. Remove from the heat and add the vanilla extract.
5. Sweeten with liquid stevia to taste and pour into serving bowls.

Nutritional Facts:

Calories: 188, Fat 10g, Cholesterol 0 mg, Carbohydrates 6g, Protein 7g

CHAPTER TWO

KETODENIC LUNCH RECIPE

Creamy Shrimp and Vegetable Curry

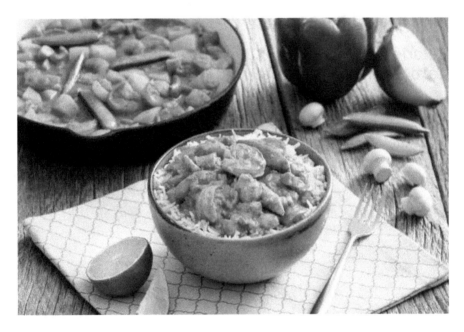

Prep Time: 9 Min | Cooking Time: 10 Min | Servings: 2

Ingredients

- 1 medium zucchini, diced
- 1 tablespoon coconut oil
- 1 cup sliced mushrooms

- 1 clove minced garlic
- ½ small yellow onion, chopped
- 12 ounces large shrimp, peeled and deveined
- 4 ounces cream cheese, softened
- 2 tablespoons shelled edamame
- 1 tablespoon soy sauce
- ¼ cup fresh chopped cilantro
- ½ teaspoon turmeric
- 1 teaspoon red curry paste
- ½ cup chicken broth

Directions

1. In an enormous skillet, heat the oil over medium heat.
2. Add zucchini, mushrooms, onion and garlic; then sauté until tender, about 6-7 minutes.
3. Arrange the shrimp in a single layer the pan and cook, 1 to 2 minutes per side, until they turn pink.
4. Add the edamame, cream cheese, soy sauce, curry paste, turmeric and broth.
5. Bake for 2 minutes or until cream cheese is melted; Adjust the seasoning to taste.
6. Pour into bowls and serve with fresh cilantro

Nutritional Facts:

Calories: 425, Fat 28g, Carbohydrates 12g, Protein 34g, Cholesterol 265 mg

Delicious Grilled Cheese

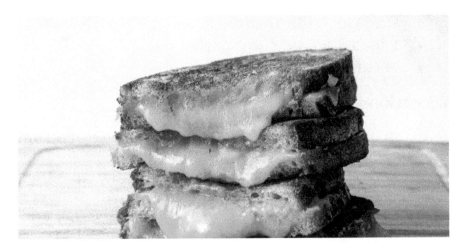

Prep Time: 10 Min | Cooking Time: 28 Min | Servings: 2

Ingredients:

- ½ cup mozzarella, shredded
- 4 cups zucchinis, shredded and drained well
- 1 egg
- 4 tablespoons parmesan, grated
- A drizzle of olive oil
- A pinch of salt and black pepper
- 1/3 cup cheddar cheese, shredded
- 1 tablespoon ghee, soft
- 1 teaspoon oregano, dried

Directions:

1. Line a baking sheet along with parchment paper and grease with oil.
2. In a portable bowl, mix the zucchini with salt, pepper, mozzarella, parmesan and oregano, mix well, form 4 squares of this mixture, place them on the baking sheet, put them in the oven at 450 degrees for 20 minutes.
3. Grease the zucchini with ghee, toss in a hot skillet over medium heat, sprinkle each square of zucchini with cheddar cheese, cook for 4 minutes per side, divide into plates and serve for lunch. Enjoy!

Nutritional Facts:

Calories: 155, Fat 10, Carbohydrates 8g, Protein 10g, fiber 6

Lemon Kale Salad

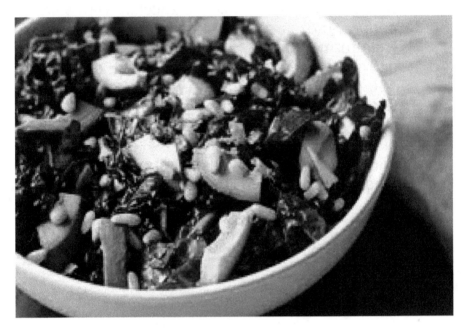

Prep Time: 10 Min | Cooking Time: 0 Min | Servings: 2

Ingredients

- ¼ cup olive oil
- 4 ounces fresh kale
- 3 tablespoons fresh lemon juice
- 2 cloves minced garlic
- 1 tablespoon fresh lemon zest
- Salt and pepper, to taste
- 2 ounces feta cheese, crumbled
- ¼ cup slivered almonds

Directions

1. Rinse the kale in freshwater; pat dry.
2. Thick stems are cut off and the leaves are cut into small pieces.
3. Put the kale in a bowl with olive oil, lemon juice, lemon zest, garlic, salt and pepper.
4. Stir to coat, then massage the cabbage for a few minutes to soften it.
5. Add almonds and feta cheese and toss to combine.

Nutritional Facts:

Calories: 431, Fat 40g, Carbohydrates 9g, Protein 10g, Cholesterol 25 mg

Loaded Cobb Salad

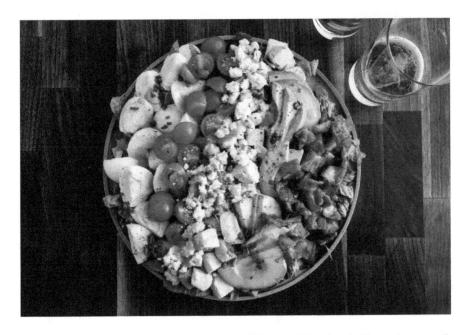

Prep Time: 11 Min | Cooking Time: 5 Min | Servings: 2

Ingredients

- 2 cups fresh baby spinach
- 4 slices bacon
- 2 large eggs, hardboiled and chopped
- Salt and pepper, to taste
- 1 small avocado, pitted and sliced
- 1 tablespoon heavy cream
- 1 tablespoon sour cream
- 1 tablespoon mayonnaise
- Pinch onion powder
- ½ teaspoon fresh chopped chives
- ¼ teaspoon fresh lemon juice

- ½ teaspoon fresh chopped parsley
- Pinch garlic powder

Directions

1. In an enormous skillet over medium heat, cook the bacon until crisp.
2. Drain on paper towels and roughly chop; set aside.
3. Divide the spinach between two salad bowls or plates.
4. Top each salad with half the eggs, avocado and bacon; Add salt and pepper.
5. In a small bowl, combine the remaining ingredients and season the salads to serve.

Nutritional Facts:

Calories: 355, Fat 30g, Carbohydrates 9g, Protein 14g, Cholesterol 220 mg

Lunch Cauliflower Salad

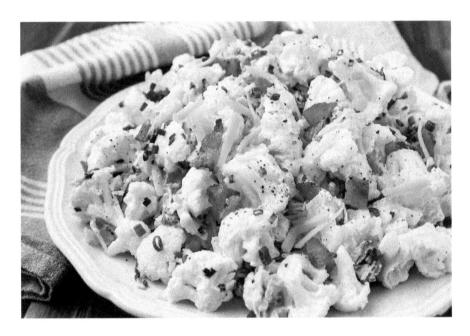

Prep Time: 10 Min | Cooking Time: 43 Min | Servings: 4

Ingredients:

- A pinch of salt and black pepper
- 1 cauliflower head, florets separated
- 3 garlic cloves, minced
- Juice of 1 lemon
- 5 tablespoons olive oil
- 2 tablespoons walnuts, chopped
- 1 tablespoon green onions, chopped

- 1 small avocado, peeled pitted and cubed

Directions:

1. Spread the cauliflower florets out on a lined baking sheet, drizzle with half of the oil, season with salt, pepper and sprinkle with garlic.
2. Toss the cauliflower, put it in the oven and bake at 425 degrees for 45 minutes.
3. Transfer the cauliflower to a salad bowl, add the nuts, lemon juice, avocado, chives and the rest of the oil, toss and serve for lunch. Enjoy!

Nutritional Facts:

Calories: 200, Fat 4g, Carbohydrates 11g, Protein 7g, fiber 6

Lunch Salmon Mix

Prep Time: 1 hour | Cooking Time: 20 Min | Servings: 4

Ingredients:

- 2 Portobello mushroom caps, sliced
- 4 salmon fillets, boneless
- 4 baby bok choy
- 1 green onion, chopped
- 1 tablespoon sesame seeds, toasted
- 1 tablespoon olive oil
- 1 teaspoon sesame oil
- 1 tablespoon coconut aminos
- 1 teaspoon ginger, grated
- A pinch of salt and black pepper
- Juice of ½ lemon

Directions:

1. In an enormous bowl, combine the salmon with olive oil, aminos, sesame oil, ginger, salt, pepper and lemon juice, mix, cover and refrigerate 1 now.
2. Spot the salmon fillets on a lined baking sheet, add the sliced mushrooms and bok choy, put it in the oven and bake at 400 degrees for 20 minutes.
3. Divide everything between plates, sprinkle with green onion and sesame seeds and serve for lunch.

Nutritional Facts:

Calories: 261, Fat 4, Carbohydrates 15g, Protein 7g,
fiber 6

Meatball Marinara Bake

Prep Time: 13 Min | Cooking Time: 30 Min | Servings: 8

Ingredients

- 4 large eggs
- 1½ pounds 80 percent lean ground beef
- 1 cup grated parmesan cheese
- 2 tablespoons almond flour
- ¼ cup diced yellow onion
- 2 cloves minced garlic
- 1 tablespoon olive oil
- Salt and pepper, to taste
- 2 cups no-sugar-added marinara sauce
- Fresh chopped parsley, to serve
- 2 cups shredded mozzarella cheese

Directions

1. Warm the oven to 350 degrees and grease a 9x9-inch baking dish with cooking spray.
2. In an enormous bowl, combine the meat, eggs, Parmesan, onion, almond flour and garlic.
3. Flavor with pepper and salt; then mix and form 16 meatballs by hand.
4. Grease an enormous skillet and heat over high heat; add the meatballs.

5. Brown the meatballs on all sides for 3 to 5 minutes, until golden brown.
6. Pour the marinara sauce into the pan and add the meatballs.
7. Garnish with grated mozzarella and bake for 20 minutes.
8. Place the pan under the grill for 2 minutes to brown the cheese.
9. Garnish with parsley to serve.

Nutritional Facts:

Calories: 356, Fat 23g, Carbohydrates 4g, Protein 29g, Cholesterol 176 mg

Mexican Chicken Lunch Mix

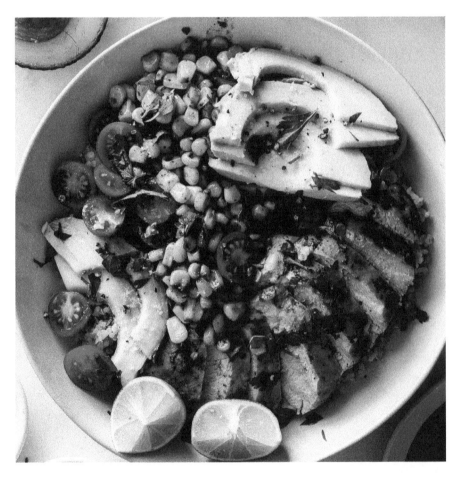

Prep Time: 10 Min | Cooking Time: 21 Min | Servings: 4

Ingredients:

- 1 cup keto enchilada sauce
- 4 chicken breast halves, skinless, boneless and cut into strips
- Cauliflower rice, cooked for serving
- ¼ cup yellow onion, chopped
- 4 ounces canned green chilies, chopped
- ¼ cup water

Directions:

1. Warm a skillet over medium-high heat; add the chicken strips and sauté for 5 to 6 minutes.
2. Add the onion, water, enchilada sauce and chilies, stir, cover the pan, lower the heat to medium and cook for 15 minutes.
3. Divide the cauliflower between plates, top each with the chicken mixture and serve for lunch.

Nutritional Facts:

Calories: 251, Fat 4, Carbohydrates 14g, Protein 7g, fiber 8

Salmon Rolls

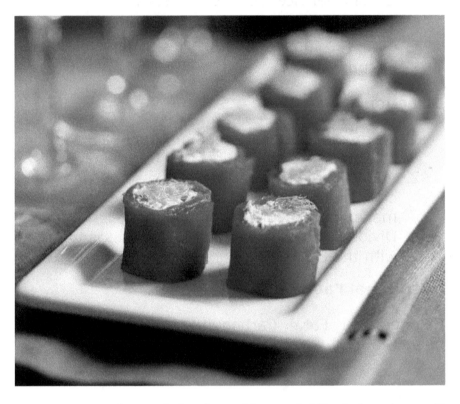

Prep Time: 10 Min | Cooking Time: 0 Min | Servings: 3

Ingredients:

- 5 ounce canned salmon, dried and flaked
- 3 nori sheets
- One red bell pepper, cut into thin strips
- 1 small cucumber, cut into thin strips
- 1 small avocado, pitted, peeled and cut into thin strips
- 1 spring onion, chopped

- Coconut aminos for serving
- 1 tablespoon mayonnaise

Directions:

1. Place the nori sheets on a cutting board, divide the salmon, pepper, avocado, cucumber, onion and mayonnaise, roll well, cut each roll into 2 pieces and serve with the Coconut aminos on the side.

Nutritional Facts:

Calories: 200, Fat 4, Carbohydrates 11g, Protein 6g, fiber 7

Shrimp and Asparagus Salad

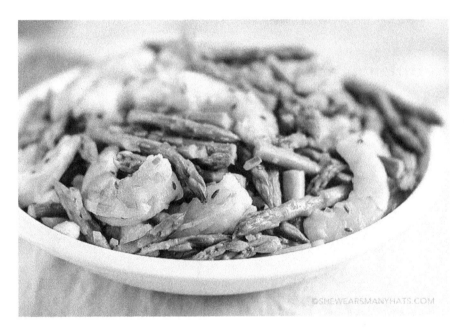

Prep Time: 11 Min | Cooking Time: 7 Min | Servings: 2

Ingredients:

- 1 teaspoon thyme, dried
- 1 pound shrimp, peeled and deveined
- 2 garlic cloves, minced
- A pinch of salt and black pepper
- 1 teaspoon basil, dried
- 2 bunches asparagus, trimmed and halved
- 2 teaspoons sweet paprika
- 1 teaspoon olive oil

40

- A handful basil, torn
- 4 cups lettuce leaves, torn
- 1 small red onion, chopped
- 2 tablespoons water
- 1/3 cup coconut cream
- 1 avocado, peeled, pitted and cubed
- 1 teaspoon lemon juice

Directions:

1. Over medium heat, heat a pan with the oil, add the shrimp, thyme, garlic, basil, salt, pepper, paprika and asparagus, mix and cook for 5 minutes.
2. In a handy bowl, combine the shrimp and asparagus with lettuce, basil, onion, avocado, coconut cream, lemon juice and water, mix well and serve for lunch.

Nutritional Facts:

Calories: 251, Fat 4, Carbohydrates 15g, Protein 7g, fiber 7

Zucchini Broccoli Chicken Sliders

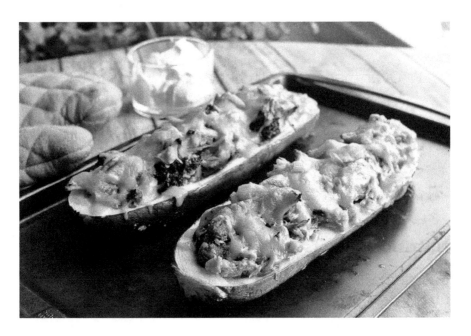

Prep Time: 10 Min | Cooking Time: 44 Min | Servings: 4

Ingredients

- 6 oz. Rotisserie Chicken, shredded
- 2 large zucchinis - hallowed out
- 3 oz. Cheddar Cheese, shredded
- 1 cup Broccoli
- 1 stalk Green Onion
- 2 tbsp. Sour Cream
- Salt and Pepper, to taste

- 2 tbsp. Butter – melted

Directions

1. Preheat the oven to 400 F.
2. Cut the zucchini in half lengthwise and collect most of the zucchini until the skin is about 1 cm thick. Pour the butter over each zucchini. Add salt and pepper. Place the zucchini in the oven and bake for about 20 minutes.
3. While the zucchini cooks, shred the chicken. Break the florets of broccoli into small parts, and mix them with sour cream. Add salt and pepper.
4. When the zucchini is cooked, including the chicken and broccoli filling. Sprinkle cheddar cheese over each pan of zucchini and cook for another 10 to 15 minutes or until cheese is melted.
5. Top with chopped green onion and enjoy with keto mayonnaise. Serve immediately and enjoy your food!

Nutritional Facts:

Calories: 145, Fat 33.98g, Carbohydrates 5g, Protein 30g

CHAPTER THREE

KETOGENIC DINNER RECIPE

Keto zucchini slice

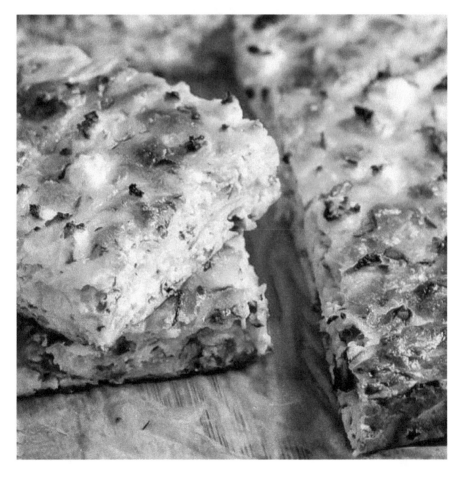

Prep Time: 16 Min | Cooking Time: 30 Min | Servings: 10

Ingredients

- 2/5 small Onion diced
- 2/5 tablespoon Salted Butter
- 4/5 cloves Garlic crushed
- 4/5 ounces Baby Spinach roughly chopped
- 4/5 large Zucchini approx. 600g/21oz
- 1/5 cup Cheddar Cheese shredded
- 2/5 cup Almond Flour
- 1/5 cup Feta Cheese crumbled
- 1/10 cup Heavy Cream
- 2/5 teaspoon Baking Powder
- 1/5 teaspoon Pepper ground
- 2/5 teaspoon salt
- 2 large Eggs

Directions

1. Preheat the oven to 180 ° C.
2. Spot the butter, onion, and garlic in a small saucepan and sauté over medium heat until the onion becomes translucent.
3. Coarsely grate the zucchini, place them on a clean towel or muslin cloth and wring out as much liquid as possible.
4. In an enormous bowl, add the onion mixture, zucchini, spinach, cheddar cheese, half the feta cheese, baking powder, almond flour, salt, and pepper. Blend them together.
5. Include the eggs and cream and mix well.
6. Prepare an 8 x 12-inch baking dish by lining it with parchment paper.

7. Empty the zucchini mixture into the pan and smooth.
8. Sprinkle with remaining feta cheese.
9. Bake for 25 to 35 minutes until an inserted skewer is golden and clean.
10. Let cool for 15 minutes before spreading and enjoying.

Nutritional Facts

Calories 76, Carbohydrates 2g, Protein: 4g, Fat: 6g, Cholesterol: 47mg

Lamb Burgers

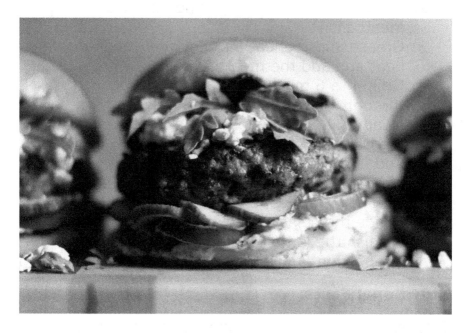

Prep Time: 7 Min | Cooking Time: 15 Min | Servings: 2

Ingredients

- 2 teaspoons dried rosemary
- 10 ounces ground lamb
- 1 teaspoon dried thyme
- Salt and pepper, to taste
- 1 clove minced garlic
- 1 teaspoon olive oil
- ¼ cup sour cream
- 1 teaspoon dried onion flakes
- 12 ounces fresh baby spinach
- 2 ounces goat cheese

Directions

1. In a large bowl, combine the lamb, rosemary, thyme, garlic, salt, and pepper.
2. Mix well, then shape by hand into two meatballs.
3. Grease and preheat a skillet over medium-high heat and add the meatballs.
4. Grill, 4 to 6 minutes per side, until cooked through.
5. Meanwhile, in an enormous skillet, heat oil over medium-high heat.
6. Add spinach and sauté until wilted, about 1 to 2 minutes; then stir in sour cream and season with salt and pepper.
7. Divide the spinach between two plates and garnish the lamb patties with goat cheese and dried onion flakes to serve.

Nutritional Facts:

Calories: 528, Fat 35, Carbohydrates 12g, Protein 35g, Cholesterol 128 mg

Marinara Poached Cod

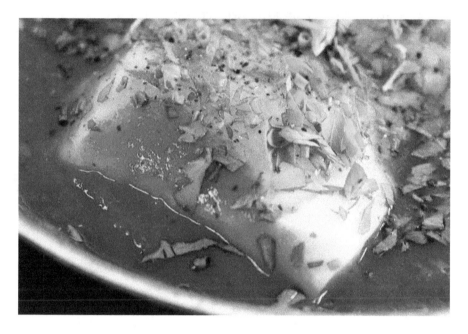

Prep Time: 7 Min | Cooking Time: 15 Min | Servings: 2

Ingredients

- ½ cup sugar-free marinara sauce
- 2 tablespoons olive oil
- 1 tablespoon fresh chopped basil
- 3 small bay leaves
- 2 cloves minced garlic
- 2 cups green beans, sliced
- Salt and pepper, to taste
- 1 teaspoon coconut oil

- Two 8-ounce cod fillets

Directions

1. In a saucepan, heat the olive oil, marinara sauce, basil, and garlic over medium heat.
2. Add bay leaves, salt, and pepper and simmer for 5 minutes.
3. Lower the heat and add the cod fillets.
4. Cover and cook for 10 minutes, turning the fish once halfway through cooking.
5. In another skillet, brown the green beans in the coconut oil until tender.
6. When the cod is cooked, serve with the green beans.

Nutritional Facts:

Calories: 403, Fat 22, Carbohydrates 8g, Protein 39g, Cholesterol 86 mg

Pan-Seared Pork Chops with Apple

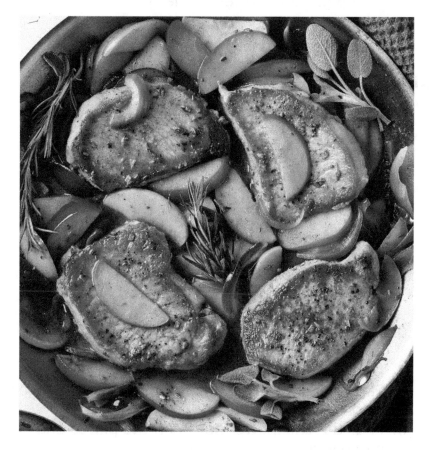

Prep Time: 11 Min | Cooking Time: 20 Min | Servings: 2

Ingredients

- ½ teaspoon dried thyme

- Two 6-ounce boneless pork loin chops
- Salt and pepper, to taste
- 2 sprigs of fresh rosemary
- ½ cup sliced apple
- 1 tablespoon olive oil
- 2 tablespoons heavy cream
- ¼ cup grated parmesan cheese
- 2 cups cauliflower, chopped
- 2 tablespoons unsalted butter

Directions

1. Season the pork chops with thyme, salt, and pepper.
2. In an enormous skillet, heat the oil over high heat and add the pork; brown on both sides.
3. Lower the heat, then decorate the pork with apples and rosemary.
4. Cover & cook for six to eight minutes until cooked through.
5. Meanwhile, place the steamer in a medium saucepan with 1 inch of water; add the cauliflower.
6. Boil water and steam the cauliflower for 8 minutes until tender.
7. Drain the cauliflower and mash it with the Parmesan, butter, and cream in a bowl; Season with salt and pepper to taste.
8. Pour the cauliflower puree on the plates and serve with the pork chops.

Nutritional Facts:

Calories: 582, Fat 43, Carbohydrates 6g, Protein 39g, Cholesterol 155 mg

Parmesan Meatballs with Zoodles

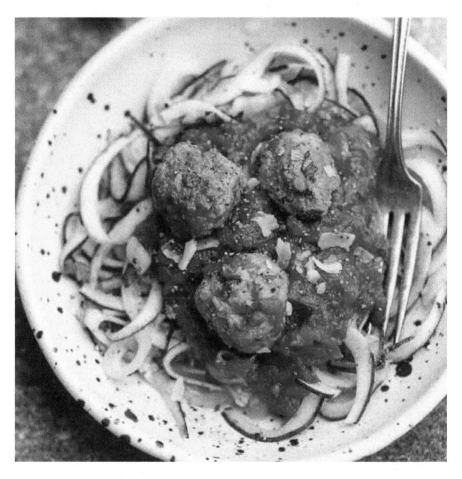

Prep Time: 9 Min | Cooking Time: 16 Min | Servings: 2

Ingredients

- ¼ cup plus 2 tablespoons grated parmesan cheese
- ½ pound 80 percent lean ground beef
- 2 tablespoons almond flour
- 1 large egg
- 1 clove minced garlic
- 1 tablespoon fresh chopped parsley
- Salt and pepper, to taste
- 1 tablespoon fresh chopped basil
- ½ cup sugar-free pasta sauce
- 1 medium zucchini, spiralized

Directions

1. In an enormous bowl, combine the beef, ¼ cup of Parmesan, almond flour, garlic, and egg.
2. Flavor with pepper and salt, then mix well by hand into 1-inch balls.
3. Grease an enormous skillet with cooking spray and heat over high heat.
4. Include the meatballs and brown on all sides; lower the heat and add the pasta sauce and basil.
5. Simmer, covered, for 10 minutes, spiralizing the zucchini noodles.
6. Cook the noodles in a greased pan over medium heat for 2 minutes until cooked through.
7. The meatballs should be served on a bed of zucchini noodles and pour into the excess sauce.
8. Dress with the remaining two tbsp of Parmesan and freshly grated parsley for serving.

Nutritional Facts:

Calories: 381, Fat 24, Carbohydrates 6g, Protein 32g, Cholesterol 177 mg

Pork Carnitas

Prep Time: 5 Min | Cooking Time: 4 hours and 1o minutes | Servings: 4

Ingredients:

- 2 tablespoons avocado oil
- 1 cup water
- 4 pounds pork roast
- ½ teaspoon black pepper
- 2 teaspoon juniper berries
- 1 teaspoon thyme
- 1 teaspoon Himalayan sea salt

Directions:

1. Commence by preheating the oven to 300 degrees Fahrenheit.
2. Then take a casserole dish, put it on the stove, and set the flame to medium. Add avocado oil to the jar.
3. While the pan is heating, take the roast pork and sprinkle it with sea salt. Then place the roast in the casserole dish and brown the sides for a minute on each side.
4. Turn off the heat once the roast is golden brown. Add the water, thyme, juniper berries, and black pepper to the pot, then cover. Spot the pan in the preheated oven and cook the roast for 3.5 hours. Flip the roast every half-hour, so the flavors really penetrate all areas of the meat.

5. Remove the roast after 3.5 hours (leave the oven on), let it stand for 10 minutes, then separate the meat with two forks. After pulling all the meat, return the pan to the oven for 30 minutes. Remove the pot and enjoy!

Nutritional Facts:

Calories 317, Carbs .5g, Fat 14.5g, Protein 43g

Salmon with Avocado Lime Puree

Prep Time: 10 Min | Cooking Time: 21 Min | Servings: 2

Ingredients

- 2 tablespoons fresh chopped cilantro
- 1 cup cauliflower, chopped
- 1 clove minced garlic
- 1 medium avocado
- Salt and pepper, to taste
- 2 tablespoons canned coconut milk
- 2 tablespoons diced red onion
- 1 teaspoon coconut oil
- 1 tablespoon fresh lime juice
- Two 6-ounce boneless salmon fillets

Directions

1. Spot the cauliflower in a food processor and mix it into rice-like grains.
2. Grease a large skillet and heat over low heat; then add the cauliflower, cilantro, and garlic.
3. Flavor with pepper and salt and cook, covered, 8 minutes, until tender.
4. In a blender, combine the avocado, coconut milk, and lemon juice and season with salt and pepper.

5. Mix until you obtain a homogeneous and creamy mixture; then set aside.
6. In an enormous skillet, heat the coconut oil over medium heat.
7. Season the salmon with salt and pepper.
8. Include the salmon in the pan and cook, 4 to 5 minutes per side, until cooked through.
9. Pour the cauliflower on the plates, garnish with a salmon fillet and garnish with the avocado and lime puree and chopped red onion.

Nutritional Facts:

Calories: 411, Fat 24, Carbohydrates 9g, Protein 40g, Cholesterol 80 mg

Soy Glazed Chicken

Prep Time: 37 Min | Cooking Time: 20 Min | Servings: 2

Ingredients

- 2 tablespoons fresh lemon juice
- ¼ cup soy sauce
- 1 teaspoon fresh grated ginger
- 1 jalapeño pepper, seeded and minced
- 2 cloves minced garlic
- 4 boneless chicken thighs, skin on
- 2 cups green beans, sliced
- 2 tablespoons olive oil

Directions

1. In an enormous bowl, combine the soy sauce, lemon juice, ginger, garlic, and jalapeño pepper.
2. Add the chicken thighs and marinate for 30 minutes.
3. Warm the oil in an enormous skillet over medium heat.
4. Include the chicken thighs and cook for 8 to 10 minutes per side.
5. Cook the green beans in another pan over medium-high heat until golden brown.
6. Serve the chicken with green beans.

Nutritional Facts:

Calories: 782, Fat 54, Carbohydrates 5g, Protein 64g, Cholesterol 365 mg

CHAPTER FOUR

APPETIZERS, SIDES AND SNACKS

Keto Corndog Muffins

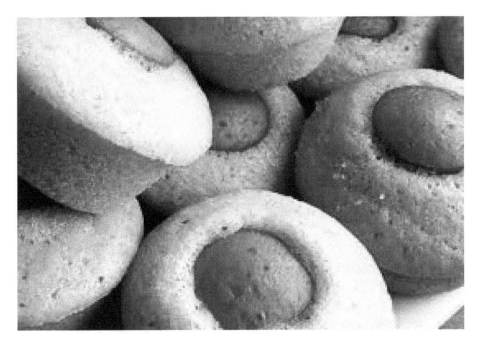

Prep Time: 13 Min | Cooking Time: 15 Min | Servings: 3

Ingredients

- 1/2 cup Almond Flour

- 1 large Egg
- 1/2 cup Flaxseed Meal
- 1/4 cup Butter, melted
- 1/3 cup Sour Cream
- 1/4 cup Coconut Milk
- 1 tbsp. Psyllium Husk Powder
- 3 tbsp. Swerve Sweetener
- 1/4 tsp. Baking Powder
- Salt
- 3 hot dogs

Directions

1. Preheat the oven to 375 F.
2. Combine the dry ingredients in a bowl. Add the egg, coconut milk, sour cream, and butter and mix well.
3. Divide the batter into the muffin slots. Cut the sausages into three pieces and place them in the center of each muffin pan.
4. Cook for 12 minutes. Then broil for two minutes until the top is golden. Let the muffins cool.

Nutritional Facts:

Calories: 80, Fat 6.9, Carbohydrates 0.6g, Protein 2.5g

Keto Flax Tortillas

Prep Time: 13 Min | Cooking Time: 10 Min | Servings: 4

Ingredients

- 1 cup Flax Seed Meal
- 1 cup + 2 tbsp. Water
- 2 tbsps. Psyllium Husk Powder
- 1/2 tsp. Curry Powder
- 2 tsps. Olive Oil
- 1/4 tsp. Xanthan Gum
- Extra Olive Oil
- Coconut Flour

Directions

1. Combine all the dry ingredients together, and afterward, add the water and 2 tbsp. Oil. Mix until the dough forms. Let it stand an hour without the lid.
2. Divide the tortilla into three portions if hand-rolled. Press down on your hand and sprinkle coconut flour on the face of the tortilla, and roll until fine.
3. Warm the oil over medium-high heat in a skillet and fry until desired.

Nutritional Facts:

Calories: 165, Fat 19.3g, Carbohydrates 0.5g, Protein 6.5g

Lime Cauliflower Rice

Prep Time: 13 Min | Cooking Time: 15 Min | Servings: 4

Ingredients:

- Juice of 2 limes
- 1 tablespoon ghee, melted
- A pinch of salt and black pepper
- 1 tablespoon cilantro, chopped
- 1 and ½ cups veggie stock
- 1 cup cauliflower rice

Directions:

1. Heat a pan with clarified butter over medium-high heat, add the cauliflower rice, stir and cook for 5 minutes.
2. Add lemon juice, salt, pepper, and broth, mix, bring to a boil, and cook for 10 minutes.
3. Add the cilantro, mix, divide between plates and serve as a garnish.

Nutritional Facts:

Calories: 181, Fat 2g, Carbohydrates 9g, Protein 6g, fibers 5

Low-Carb Chia Bars

Prep Time: 15 Min | Cooking Time: 40 Min | Servings: 5

Ingredients

- 1 cup Ice Water
- 3 oz. Shredded Cheddar Cheese
- 1/2 cup Chia Seeds
- 2 tbsps. Psyllium Husk Powder
- 2 tbsps. Olive Oil
- 1/4 tsp. Xanthan Gum
- 1/4 tsp. Garlic Powder
- 1/4 tsp. Onion Powder
- 1/4 tsp. Paprika
- Salt and Pepper
- 1/4 tsp. Oregano

Directions

1. Preheat the oven to 375F.
2. Crush the chia seeds. Add the dry ingredients and crush the chia seeds in a bowl. Add olive oil and mix with the dry ingredients.
3. Spout the water into the bowl and mix until paste forms. Add the grated cheddar cheese and mix the cheese with the batter. Spot on a baking sheet and let stand. Spread the dough thinly in the pan.
4. Cook for 30 minutes.
5. Take it away from heat and cut it into individual pieces. Return the chia bars to the oven and

bake for 5 minutes or until the cookies are crisp.
6. Serve immediately and enjoy!

Nutritional Facts:

Calories: 30, Fat 2.5, Carbohydrates 0g, Protein 1.3g

Mini Caprese Skewers

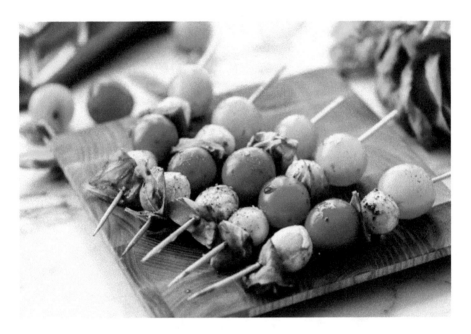

Prep Time: 10 minutes | Cooking Time: 0 Min | Servings: 4

Ingredients

- 4 ounces fresh mozzarella
- 16 cherry tomatoes
- Salt and pepper, to taste
- 8 large basil leaves, torn in half
- 2 tablespoons balsamic vinegar
- 2 tablespoons olive oil

Directions

1. Split the cherry tomatoes into halve and cut the mozzarella into cubes.
2. Using the wooden chopsticks, make skewers with two tomato halves, two mozzarella cubes and a basil leaf cut in half.
3. Put the skewers on a plate or platter.
4. Season with olive oil and balsamic vinegar; then season with salt and pepper to serve.

Nutritional Facts:

Calories: 159, Fat 14g, Carbohydrates 3g, Protein 5g, Cholesterol 23 mg

Pesto Bread Strips

Prep Time: 10 minutes | Cooking Time: 20 Min
| Servings: 8

Ingredients

- ¼ cup coconut flour
- ½ cup almond flour
- 1 teaspoon baking powder
- ½ teaspoon salt
- 1 large egg, whisked well
- ½ teaspoon garlic powder
- 1½ cups shredded mozzarella cheese
- 2 ounces pesto sauce
- 5 tablespoons unsalted butter, softened

Directions

1. Warm the oven to 350 degrees and line a baking sheet with parchment paper.
2. In a portable bowl, combine the almond flour, coconut flour, baking powder, garlic powder and salt.
3. In a small saucepan, melt the cheese and butter over low heat and mix well.
4. Remove the cheese and butter from the heat and add the mixture to the dry ingredients to form a paste.
5. Roll the dough in the middle of two sheets of parchment paper, until it is ¼ inch thick.
6. Spread the pesto over the pasta; then cut it into 1 inch strips.

7. Place the bread strips on the baking sheet and brush them out with the egg.
8. Bake for 15 to 20 minutes, until golden brown; then serve hot.

Nutritional Facts:

Calories: 226, Fat 20g, Carbohydrates3, Protein 8g, Cholesterol 61 mg

Simple Crackers

Prep Time: 10 minutes | Cooking Time: 15 Min | Servings: 6

Ingredients:

- Salt and black pepper to the taste
- ½ teaspoon baking powder
- 1 and ¼ cups almond flour
- 3 tablespoons ghee
- 1 garlic clove, minced
- ¼ teaspoon basil, dried
- 2 tablespoons basil pesto

Directions:

1. In a portable bowl, combine the salt, pepper, baking powder, almond flour, garlic, basil, pesto and ghee and mix the dough with your fingers.
2. Spread this dough on a lined baking sheet, place in the oven at 325 degrees F, bake for 17 minutes, cut into medium cookies when it's cold enough, and serve as a snack.

Nutritional Facts:

Calories: 200, Fat 20g, Carbohydrates 4g, Protein 7g, fiber 1

Tuna Cakes

Prep Time: 10 minutes | Cooking Time: 18 Min | Servings: 12

Ingredients:

- 3 eggs
- 15 ounces canned tuna, drained and flaked
- A drizzle of olive oil
- 1 teaspoon parsley, dried
- 1 teaspoon garlic powder
- ½ cup red onion, chopped
- Salt and black pepper to the taste

Directions:

1. In a portable bowl, mix the tuna with the salt, pepper, parsley, onion, garlic powder and eggs, mix and form medium patties with this mixture.
2. Heat a pan with the oil over medium-high heat, add the cakes, toss and cook for 4 minutes per side.
3. Arrange the meatballs on a serving plate and serve as an appetizer.

Nutritional Facts:

Calories: 160, Fat 2g, Carbohydrates 6g, Protein 6g, fibers 4

Zucchini Chips

Prep Time: 11 minutes | Cooking Time: 3 hours | Servings: 8

Ingredients:

- 3 zucchinis, thinly sliced
- Salt and black pepper to the taste
- 2 tablespoons balsamic vinegar
- 2 tablespoons olive oil

Directions:

1. In a handy bowl, mix the oil with the vinegar, salt and pepper, beat well, add the zucchini slices, mix well to cover, spread them in a lined pan, put in the oven at 200 degrees, cook in oven for 3 hours, leave the fried potatoes to cool and serve as snacks.

Nutritional Facts:

Calories: 100, Fat 3g, Carbohydrates 7g, Protein 7g, fibers 3

Zucchini Spread

Prep Time: 10 minutes | Cooking Time: 6 Min | Servings: 4

Ingredients:

- 3 tablespoons veggie stock
- 4 cups zucchinis, chopped
- ¼ cup olive oil
- ½ cup lemon juice
- 4 garlic cloves, minced
- Salt and black pepper to the taste
- ¾ cup sesame seeds paste

Directions:

1. Over medium-high heat, heat a pan with half of the oil, add the zucchini and garlic, stir and cook for 2 minutes.
2. Add the broth, salt and pepper, mix and cook for another 4 minutes.
3. Transfer the zucchini to the blender, add the remaining oil, sesame paste and lemon juice, mix well, transfer to bowls and serve.

Nutritional Facts:

Calories: 140, Fat 5g, Carbohydrates 6g, Protein 7g, fibers 3

Broccoli Biscuits

Prep Time: 13 minutes | Cooking Time: 25 Min | Servings: 12

Ingredients:

- 1 and ½ cup almond flour
- 4 cups broccoli florets
- 1 teaspoon sweet paprika
- 2 eggs
- Salt and black pepper to the taste
- ¼ cup olive oil
- ½ teaspoon baking soda
- 1 teaspoon garlic powder
- 2 cups cheddar cheese, grated
- ½ teaspoon apple cider vinegar

Directions:

1. In your food processor, combine the broccoli with salt and pepper, beat well and transfer to a bowl.
2. Add flour, paprika, salt, pepper, eggs, oil, cheese, garlic powder, vinegar and baking soda.
3. Mix them together and form 12 meatballs, place on a baking sheet, place in oven at 375 ° F, bake for 20 minutes, place on platter and serve as a snack.

Nutritional Facts:

Calories: 183, Fat 12g, Carbohydrates 8g, Protein 4g, fibers 2

Cream Cheese and Olives Bombs

Prep Time: 10 minutes | Cooking Time: 0 Min | Servings: 6

Ingredients:

- Salt and black pepper to the taste
- 8 black olives, pitted and chopped
- 2 tablespoons basil pesto
- 4 ounces cream cheese
- 14 pepperoni slices, chopped

Directions:

1. In a handy bowl, mix the cream cheese with the salt, pepper, pepperoni, pesto and black olives, mix well, form balls with this mixture, place in a serving dish and serve.

Nutritional Facts:

Calories: 140, Fat 4g, Carbohydrates 14g, Protein 3g, fibers 4

Crispy Baked Onion Rings

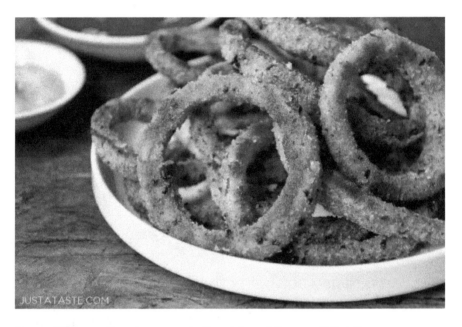

Prep Time: 5 minutes | Cooking Time: 20 Min | Servings: 4

Ingredients

- 1 cup almond flour
- 1 large yellow onion
- 1 large egg, whisked well
- ½ cup grated parmesan cheese
- 1 teaspoon paprika
- 1 teaspoon garlic powder
- ¼ teaspoon salt

Directions

1. Warm the oven to 400 degrees and line parchment paper with a baking sheet.
2. Cut the onion into ¼-inch-thick rings.
3. In a portable bowl, combine the almond flour, Parmesan, garlic powder, paprika and salt.
4. In another portable bowl, beat the egg then immerse the onion rings.
5. Dip the onion rings in the almond flour mixture; then place them in the pan.
6. Spray with cooking spray and cook, 15 to 20 minutes, until crispy and golden. Flip them in half if necessary.

Nutritional Facts:

Calories: 240, Fat 18g, Carbohydrates 11g, Protein 12g, Cholesterol 55 mg

CHAPTER FIVE

KETOGENIC DESSERT RECIPES

Easy Cinnamon Mug Cake

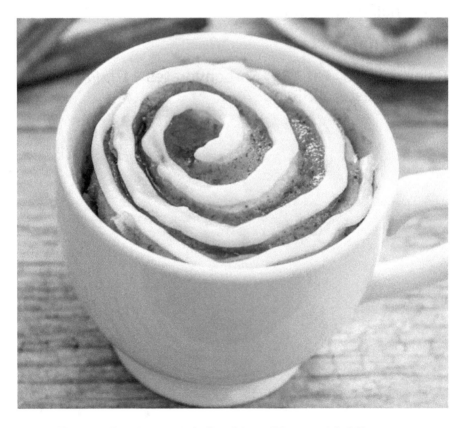

Prep Time: 5 minutes | Cooking Time: 10 Min
| Servings: 1

Ingredients

- ¾ teaspoon ground cinnamon, divided
- 2 tablespoons powdered erythritol, divided
- ¼ cup almond flour
- Pinch salt
- Sugar-free maple syrup
- ¼ teaspoon ground nutmeg
- 1 large egg
- ½ teaspoon vanilla extract
- 1 tablespoon unsalted butter, melted

Directions

1. In a small bowl, mix ½ tablespoon of erythritol with ¼ teaspoon of cinnamon and set it aside.
2. Turn on the oven and preheat to 350 degrees and grease a 4-ounce pan with cooking spray.
3. In a small bowl, combine the almond flour with the remaining erythritol, remaining cinnamon, nutmeg, and salt until combined.
4. Add egg, butter, and vanilla extract until smooth.
5. Pour the mixture into the greased plate and sprinkle with the erythritol and cinnamon mixture.
6. Bake for 12 minutes (or microwave over high heat for 1 minute) until solid
7. Drizzle with unsweetened maple syrup and serve in the baking dish

Nutritional Facts:

Calories: 349, Fat 31g, Carbohydrates 11g, Protein 13g, Cholesterol 217 mg

Easy Cookies

Prep Time: 10 Min | Cooking Time: 41 Min | Servings: 12

Ingredients:

- ¼ teaspoon cream of tartar
- 6 tablespoons stevia
- 4 egg whites
- ½ teaspoon almond extract

Directions:

1. In a portable bowl, mix the egg white with the tartar and mix with a mixer.
2. Add half of the stevia and almond extract and mix again.
3. Add the rest of the stevia, mix again and transfer everything to a piping bag.
4. Pipe out 18 cookies into a lined pan, place in the oven, and bake at 210 degrees for 40 minutes.
5. Serve them cold.

Nutritional Facts:

Calories: 190, Fat 2g, Carbohydrates 2g, Protein 2g, fibers 3

Keto Hot Cocoa

Prep Time: 10 minutes | Cooking Time: 10 Min | Servings: 4

Ingredients

- 2 tbsp. Unsweetened Cocoa Powder
- 1 1/2 Cup Unsweetened Coconut Milk
- 2 tbsp. Heavy Cream
- 1 tsp. Instant Coffee
- 1/2 tsp. Vanilla Extract
- 1 tbsp. Splenda
- 1/2 tsp. Cinnamon

Directions

1. Pour the coconut milk and cream into a saucepan over medium heat.
2. Let the milk mixture steam. Add the coffee and cinnamon. Mix well.
3. Add the cocoa powder, vanilla, and Splenda. Stir until well combined.
4. Increase the heat until it boils.
5. Once the mixture is boiling, adjust the heat to a low level and continue to stir.
6. Serve immediately and enjoy!

Nutritional Facts:

Calories: 206, Fat 18g, Carbohydrates 13g, Protein 2g

Keto Tropical Smoothie

Prep Time: 15 minutes | Cooking Time: 0 Min | Servings: 4

Ingredients

- 1/4 cup Sour Cream
- 3/4 cup Unsweetened Coconut Milk
- 2 tbsp. Golden Flaxseed Meal
- 1/2 tsp. Mango Extract
- 1 tbsp. Olive Oil
- 6 Ice Cubes
- 1/4 tsp. Banana Extract
- 20 drops Liquid Stevia
- 1/4 tsp. Blueberry Extract

Directions

1. Add all the ingredients to a blender. Permit the mixture to sit for at least 3 minutes so that the flax flour soaks up. Mix until you get a homogeneous mixture.
2. Serve immediately and enjoy your food!

Nutritional Facts:

Calories: 351, Fat 30.8g, Carbohydrates 3g, Protein 4.9g

Key Lime Panna Cotta

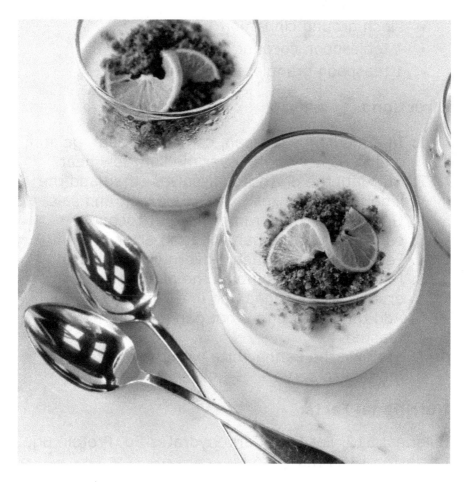

Prep Time: 10 minutes | Cooking Time: 2 Min | Servings: 4

Ingredients

- One 8-gram packet of unflavored gelatin
- 2 cups heavy cream
- ¼ cup granulated erythritol
- ½ teaspoon vanilla extract
- 4 key limes, juiced and zested
- Pinch salt
- ¼ cup almond flour
- Pinch ground cinnamon
- 1 tablespoon coconut oil
- 1 teaspoon granulated erythritol

Directions

1. In a medium saucepan, combine cream, gelatin, and ¼ cup erythritol over medium-low heat.
2. Stir until the erythritol dissolves; then add the lime juice, lime zest, vanilla extract, and salt.
3. Grease four small ramekins with coconut oil, then pour the panna cotta batter.
4. Let it cool for 4-6 hours overnight until solid.
5. Before serving, combine the almond flour, erythritol, and cinnamon in a small bowl.
6. Add the mixture to a hot pan and simmer until toasted.
7. Sprinkle the panna cotta with the toasted mixture to serve.

Nutritional Facts:

Calories: 512, Fat 51g, Carbohydrates 9g, Protein 6g, Cholesterol 164 mg

Lemon Cupcakes

Prep Time: 11 Min | Cooking Time: 30 Min | Servings: 4

Ingredients:

- 1 teaspoon baking powder
- 2 and ½ cups almond flour
- 1 cup stevia
- 2 tablespoons ghee, melted
- 2 tablespoons lemon zest, grated
- 3 eggs
- 2 teaspoons lemon extract
- 1 cup almond milk
- 1 tablespoon vanilla extract
- 3 tablespoons coconut cream
- 1 teaspoon lemon juice

Directions:

1. In a portable bowl, combine the flour with the baking powder, stevia, lemon zest, ghee, eggs, almond milk, lemon extract, vanilla, lemon juice, and cream. Whisk well, pour into a muffin pan, place in the oven and bake at 350 degrees F for 30 minutes.
2. Serve the cupcakes cold. Enjoy!

Nutritional Facts:

Calories: 332, Fat 14g, Carbohydrates 6g, Protein 8g, fibers 5

Lemon Jell-O Cake

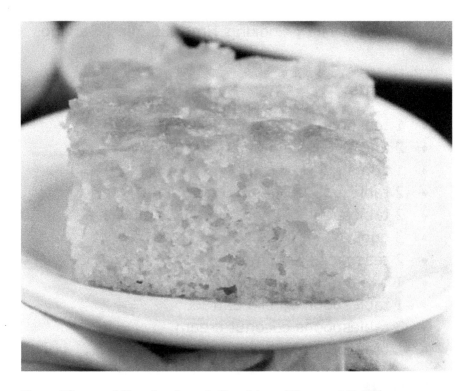

Prep Time: 15 minutes | Cooking Time: 15 Min
| Servings: 4

Ingredients

- 1 teaspoon monk fruit and erythritol blend
  sweetener, 1:1 sweetness
- 1 cup unsalted pecans
- of sugar
- Pinch salt
- ½ teaspoon ground cinnamon
- 1 tablespoon unsalted butter, melted

- ⅔ cup boiling water
- One 0.3-ounce packet sugar-free lemon Jell-O powder
- One 8-ounce package of cream cheese, softened
- 1 teaspoon fresh lemon zest
- 2 tablespoons fresh lemon juice

Directions

1. Turn on the oven and warm to 350 degrees, and grease a 6 x 6-inch baking dish with butter.
2. Place the nuts, monk fruit sweetener, erythritol, cinnamon, and salt in a food processor.
3. Stir the mixture until it has a consistency similar to a crumb; then add the melted butter until blended.
4. Press the mixture into the prepared pan.
5. Bake for approximately 15 minutes until dry to the touch and golden brown; then refrigerate for 15 minutes.
6. In a medium bowl, combine the gelatin powder with the boiling water and stir until dissolved.
7. Add the cream cheese, lemon juice, and lemon zest, then mix until smooth.
8. Pour the mixture into the base and let it cool overnight until it is solid; cut into 4 squares to serve.

Nutritional Facts:

Calories: 404, Fat 40g, Carbohydrates 7g, Protein 7g, Cholesterol 70 mg

Matcha Cake

Prep Time: 13 Min | Cooking Time: 37 Min | Servings: 4

Ingredients:

- 2 teaspoons coconut flour
- 16 ounces cream cheese
- ½ cup swerve
- 2 teaspoons coconut cream
- 2 eggs
- ½ teaspoon vanilla extract
- 1 tablespoon matcha powder

Directions:

1. In a portable bowl, mix the cream cheese with the flour, tower, vanilla, coconut cream, matcha powder, and eggs, beat well, and spout into a greased spring mold.
2. Put it in the oven and bake at 350 degrees for 35 minutes.
3. Serve cold.

Nutritional Facts:

Calories: 350, Fat 12g, Carbohydrates 6g, Protein 8g, fibers 5

Mint Chocolate Chip Ice Cream

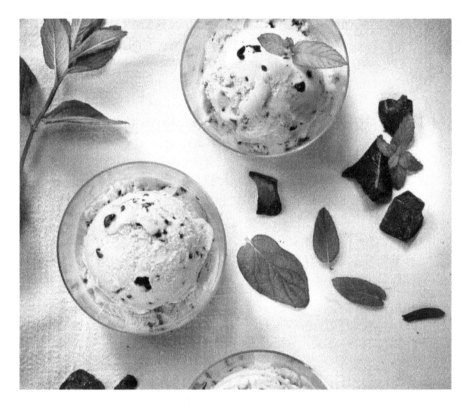

Prep Time: 20 minutes | Cooking Time: 0 Min | Servings: 8

Ingredients

- ¼ cup heavy cream
- 2 cups canned coconut milk, unsweetened
- ¾ cup powdered erythritol

- 1 teaspoon vanilla extract
- ½ cup stevia-sweetened dark chocolate chips
- 1 medium avocado, pitted and chopped
- ½ teaspoon mint extract

Directions

1. Freeze the ice cream maker's drum overnight or according to the manufacturer's instructions.
2. In a food processor, mix the coconut milk, cream, erythritol, avocado, vanilla extract, and peppermint extract and blend until smooth and blended.
3. Pour the mixture into the ice cream basket and shake according to the manufacturer's instructions.
4. Pour the mixture into an airtight container, quickly stir in the chocolate chips and freeze overnight.
5. Thaw the ice cream for like 10 to 15 minutes at room temperature before picking it up for serving.

Nutritional Facts:

Calories: 189, Fat 18g, Carbohydrates 10g, Protein 3g, Cholesterol 10 mg

Neapolitan Bars

Prep Time: 20 minutes | Cooking Time: 2 hours
| Servings: 8

Ingredients

- ¼ cup Coconut Oil
- ¼ cup Butter
- ¼ cup Cream Cheese
- 1 tbsp. Cocoa Powder
- ¼ cup Sour Cream
- 1 tbsp. Erythritol
- 2 strawberries
- ½ tsp. Vanilla extract,
- 14 drops Liquid Steve

Directions

1. With the exception of the vanilla, strawberries, and cocoa powder, combine the ingredients in a blender and mix until well combined.
2. Divide among 3 bowls and add the cocoa in one, the strawberries in the other, and the vanilla in the last. Pour the chocolate mixture into a mold and freeze for 30 minutes. Pour in the layers of strawberry and vanilla and repeat.
3. Freeze for at least 1 hour. Serve and enjoy!

Nutritional Facts:

Calories: 51, Fat 5.4g, Carbohydrates 0.2g, Protein 0.3g

Pumpkin Pudding

Prep Time: 10 minutes | Cooking Time: 1 Min
| Servings: 2

Ingredients

- ¼ cup powdered erythritol
- ½ cup canned coconut milk
- 3 tablespoons canned pumpkin puree
- 1 teaspoon pumpkin pie spice
- 1 teaspoon vanilla extract
- ⅛ teaspoon xanthan gum
- Pinch ground cinnamon
- 2 tablespoons whipped cream

Directions

1. In a portable saucepan, combine the coconut milk, erythritol, pumpkin, vanilla, pumpkin pie spice, and xanthan gum over medium heat.
2. Beat continuously for 1 minute.
3. Using a spoon, pour into a bowl and let it cool for 30 minutes until solid.
4. Divide between bowls and garnish with whipped cream and cinnamon to serve.

Nutritional Facts:

Calories: 133, Fat 12g, Carbohydrates 3g, Protein 2g, Cholesterol 10 mg

Strawberries and Cream Pancakes

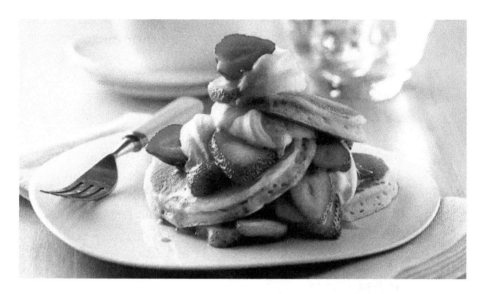

Prep Time: 10 minutes | Cooking Time: 15 Min | Servings: 2

Ingredients

- ½ teaspoon cream of tartar
- 2 large eggs, separated
- 2 ounces chopped cream cheese, divided
- ¼ teaspoon ground cinnamon
- ¼ cup sugar-free whipped cream
- ½ teaspoon vanilla extract
- 8 to 12 drops liquid stevia extract, to taste
- 1 teaspoon olive oil

- ½ cup sliced strawberries

Directions

1. In a portable bowl, beat the egg whites with a hand mixer until frothy, about 30 seconds.
2. Add cream of tartar and beat on high speed until a stiff peak is formed.
3. In a separate portable bowl, beat the egg yolks, cream cheese, vanilla extract, cinnamon, and stevia until well combined.
4. Stir in the egg whites and strawberries.
5. Pour the batter onto a griddle previously greased with ¼ cup of crepe and simmer for 4 to 5 minutes until almost cooked.
6. Gently flip the pancakes and cook until golden, about 2 minutes.
7. Transfer the pancakes onto a plate and keep them warm while you prepare the rest of the pancakes.
8. Serve hot with whipped cream on top.

Nutritional Facts:

Calories: 259, Fat 22g, Carbohydrates 6g, Protein 9g, Cholesterol 238 mg

CONCLUSION

I wanted to remind you that the ketogenic diet is always recommended for short periods of time, always better to talk with a nutritionist before starting it and to continue for a long time, always keeping blood values under control.

I hope with all my heart that the recipes designed for you, you liked them and that we had the opportunity to try them over and over again.

Choose your favorites.

Thank you for reading, and have fun with the recipes.

CPSIA information can be obtained
at www.ICGtesting.com
Printed in the USA
BVHW012330150321
602550BV00005B/631

9 781802 127096